THE ULTIMATE PRE-DIABETES MEAL PLAN

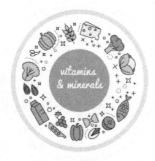

Take Charge of Your Health Reverse Prediabetes with Delicious and Nutrient-Packed Recipes| Transform Your Diet to Beat Prediabetes and Prevent Type 2 Diabetes

Dadds Dadds

Copyright © 2023 by Dadds Dadds

Can you help me to broadcast this?

I want to take a moment to say thank you for choosing my book. I want you to always remember that the power and decision to improve your health is in your hands. I understand it can be a bit challenging to forgo your favorite foods because of their negative effect on your health. However, you need to make that sacrifice before you can achieve the health goals you desire. Based on my personal experiences and the knowledge I received from experts, I am here to support you through this period. I believe you can conquer that high blood sugar, and achieve the healthy lifestyle you desire. All you need is to get the right information.

If you enjoyed this book and found it helpful, I kindly request you to leave a review. Your feedback will help anyone who has similar health challenge to discover this book. It also encourages me to continue sharing my knowledge. Thank you for being a part of this family!

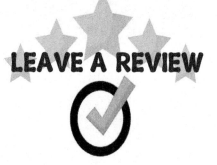

LEAVE A REVIEW

OTHER BOOKS FROM THIS AUTHOR

Do you want to explore more books from our collections? Simply scan the QR code below with your smartphone or tablet to access them.

Table of Contents

How to Utilize This Book

1. Start by reading chapter 1 and 2 to learn about the symptoms, diagnosis, risk factors, and definition of prediabetes. This will provide you with everything that you need to know about the disease, and how it affects your health.

2. In the next chapter, I explained guide on how to lower your risk of having type 2 diabetes through healthy eating and lifestyle.

3. You will find useful tips for keeping a healthy diet while arranging balanced meals, choosing foods that are good for you, and interacting with others.

4. To encourage you in this journey, I have created 3-month workout plan as bonus offer for you. Check out the interesting and successful workout regimens that suit your tastes and way of life, and jump on the challenge.

5. You will learn the connection between mental health and prediabetes, and how to cope with stress, anxiety, and depression, because of their impact on your general wellbeing.

6. There are healthy activities and suggestions provided to help manage mental health issues for prediabetes.

7. You can adjust the advice and details in this book to fit your own requirements, tastes, and way of life.

Always remember that prediabetes is a treatable illness, and that managing your health can greatly enhance your general wellbeing and lower your chance of becoming type 2 diabetes. Make the most of this book as a helpful tool to direct your path to better health and wellbeing.

"eat health nourishing foods, exercise regularly, and take proper rest. Do these and reverse prediabetes."

INTRODUCTION

Have you ever felt like your body was sending you a warning sign, telling you to take charge of your health?

Trust me, I have been through it. I found out during one of my routine check-up when my doctor hit me with the reality of my prediabetes status. The word echoed in my mind, and I was overwhelmed with fear and uncertainty. A lot of terrible thoughts flash through my mind. "Am I going to die? Is it treatable? How did this happen? These and more were questions that were bugging my mind. The most surprising thing is that I don't even take sugary foods. Somehow, I managed to pull myself together. I knew I had to act, to overcome this disease before it grows into full-blown diabetes.

There must be something out there that can help reverse this disease. I thought to myself. Then, I began to search for solution to my disease on the internet, coupled with the help of experts, what I discovered along the way was truly life-changing. I found out that food plays a great role in reversing prediabetes and regaining control over health.

During the research, I dug deep into nutrition to know more on how foods impact on the blood sugar levels and overall well-being. I tried different flavors, used fresh foods from my mini garden. I cut down on my eating out. Most importantly, I pay attention to my body.

I was amazed when I started noticing improvement in my health. The changes I made in my life made it possible. I simply created a pre-diabetes meal plan that contain whole, nutrient-rich foods, and my body responded with gratitude. Gradually, my blood sugar levels came back to normal, my energy soared, and I feel healthier. Though, it wasn't easy at first when I started the plan, but I never back down.

I want to share this life-changing process with you, to help you conquer prediabetes like me. Inside this book, I shared secrets on how to conquer prediabetes with the power of food. How to create your own nutrient-rich meal plan from scratch. I also created 80 meal plan ideas for breakfast, lunches and dinners for you. You will also find guilt-free snacks and treats, with lots of recipes that will make this journey easy and worth it.

However, this book is not just about food alone. It is about you making healthy changes to improve your general well-being. I shared practical tips for smart shopping, efficient meal prep. This will help you take charge of your health and conquer prediabetes once and for all.

Let this be the beginning of your own transformative story—a story of resilience, empowerment, and a flourishing future. Join me on this extraordinary adventure as we conquer prediabetes with the power of food, one delicious meal at a time. Together, we conquer prediabetes.

NOTE

_____

_____

_____

_____

_____

_____

_____

_____

_____

_____

_____

_____

_____

_____

_____

_____

_____

_____

_____

_____

_____

_____

_____

_____

_____

_____

_____

_____

_____

_____

_____

_____

CHAPTER 1: UNDERSTANDING PREDIABETES

I know you have a lot of questions flashing through your mind, and you want answers. Questions like "what is the meaning of prediabetes?", "What is the cause?", "what blood sugar levels is too high, normal or too low?" and why does it matters.

Prediabetes is when a person's blood sugar levels is higher than usual but not high enough to be classified as type 2 diabetes.

To simply put, Prediabetes is a stage that comes right before diabetes and is essentially your body's way of signaling, "Hey, things might not be going as smoothly as they should."

Take for instance, to have enough energy, the body uses a group of workers known as insulin to assist sugar enter the cells. Prediabetes develops when this team isn't functioning as it should. When this happens, it is a danger sign that you are at high risk of having type 2 diabetes, heart disease, and stroke.

It serves as a reminder to act in order to stop the sickness from getting worse. This book will teach you the fundamentals of prediabetes, the risk factors that go along with it, and how important food helps to control your blood sugar levels.

Understanding Blood Sugar

Your body's cells use blood sugar, commonly referred to as glucose, as their primary energy source. It originates from the food you consume, particularly from carbs. Your body converts the carbs in food into glucose, which is then released into your system. Your pancreas secretes the hormone insulin, which facilitates the uptake of glucose into your cells so they can be used as fuel.

Normal Blood Sugar Levels

The unit of measurement for blood sugar is milligrams per deciliter, or mg/dL Normal fasting blood sugar levels are usually less than 100mg/dL. Blood sugar levels is expected to be lower than 140 mg/dL two hours after eating.

Prediabetes Blood Sugar Levels

When the A1C reading falls between 5.7% and 6.4% or the fasting blood sugar level falls between 100 and 125 mg/dL, then a person is confirmed to have prediabetes. Your average blood sugar levels over the previous two to three months are measured by the A1C blood test. When your blood sugar level is higher than 180 mg/dL, two hours after eating, it is classified as higher than normal.

Risk Factors for Prediabetes

There are several things that may likely make you get prediabetes. They are:

When you are too heavy or obese (a normal body mass is said to be around 25 or lower, any body mass above 25 is considered abnormal. For men, waist circumference should be 40inches, and for women 35inches)

When you consume two much carbs than normal or overeating.

If you have any member family with type 2 diabetes

If you don't engage your body in any physical activity

If you have past record of gestational diabetes

If you have a very high blood pressure

When you have low levels of good cholesterol, or HDL,

If you possess high bad cholesterol levels, or LDL,

If you have high triglyceride

If you belong to a certain ethnic group, such as Asian American, American Indian, African American, or Hispanic/Latino.

The signs of pre-diabetes

Most times, prediabetes does not give any sign. But, for certain individuals, they experience:

A rise in thirst

Recurring urination

Excess hunger

Fatigue

hazy vision

Slow-healing wounds

Recurring infections

Complications of Prediabetes

If prediabetes is left untreated, it can result in major consequences such as:

Type 2 diabetes

Heart conditions

Stroke

renal illness / Kidney disease

Injury to the nerves

Loss of vision

Managing Prediabetes

Let me say this, it is possible to reverse prediabetes and lower the risk of acquiring type 2 diabetes by adopting certain lifestyle modifications, such as:

- **Losing Weight:** try to lose like 5-10% of your present weight. This can help improve your blood sugar levels and lower your risk of type 2 diabetes.

- **Eating a Healthy Diet:** to keep prediabetes in check, you need to maintain a healthy diet. Select meals that are low in trans and saturated fats and high in fiber. Eat mostly fruits and vegetables. Lean protein, and whole grains, but reduce (sweetened beverages, processed meals, fried foods, red meat, and full-fat dairy).

- **Getting Regular Exercise:** Try to take up at least 30 minutes moderate-intensity exercise a day, every day of the week. Exercises classified as moderate-intensity include swimming, cycling, running, and brisk walking.

- **Give Up Smoking:** The best thing you can do for your health if you smoke is to stop. Smoking raises your risk of type 2 diabetes and exacerbates prediabetes.

- **Medication:** To assist in controlling your blood sugar levels, your doctor may occasionally prescribe medication. Some medications can help reduce your chance of having type 2 diabetes.

- **Living with Prediabetes:** It might be difficult to manage prediabetes, but it's crucial to keep in mind that you're not by yourself. Many individuals with prediabetes have successfully changed their lifestyles to enhance their health.

"encourage yourself to eat healthy. Make positive changes, and create a healthier life.

NOTE

_____

_____

_____

_____

_____

_____

_____

_____

_____

_____

_____

_____

_____

NOTE

CHAPTER 2: BUILDING YOUR PERSONALIZED MEAL PLAN

Making a customized meal plan for someone with prediabetes can be a helpful first step towards improving their blood sugar and general health. To create this meal plan, you should have these at the back of your mind:

- Know how to balance carbs, proteins, and veggies you consume daily to meet your nutrient needs.
- know how to measure food portions correctly
- Learn how to plan meals ahead.

Having understood the explanation above. Below is a complete guide on how to create a meal plan that works for your unique needs and tastes:

➢ Before creating your meal plan, take a moment and examine the way you eat. For a few days, keep a record of your meal in take to see where you can make improvements. You can keep track of the kinds of food you eat, the amounts you eat, and the time you eat them. This will help you know where to begin the adjustment.

➢ The success of your meal plan depends on setting attainable and clear goals. Don't attempt to change your diet all at once. Instead, start with baby steps, and slowly improve on your set goals. For example, try to eat more fruits and vegetables, and consume less sugar-filled beverages, or include more whole grains in your dishes.

➢ Your calorie needs are influenced by a number of variables, some of them are your age, gender, degree of exercise, and present weight. To find out how many calories you should be consuming, speak with a certified dietitian or other healthcare provider. This will make sure that the meals on your menu will provide you enough energy to get through the day.

However, here is calorie consumption per day based on age, weight, and gender. You may require more calorie or less. This is why it is important to see your doctor for recommendation.

AGE	MEN	WOMEN
18 - 25	2400 - 3000	1800 – 2400
26 - 50	2200 - 3000	1800 – 2400
51 - 75	2000 - 2800	1600 – 2200
76+	2000 - 2400	1600 – 2000

➤ Pay attention to nutrient-rich foods that promote healthy blood sugar regulation and general well-being. Ensure to include them in your dishes. These foods are listed below:

a. Go for vibrant fruits with low glycemic index (GI), such citrus, apples, pears, and berries.

Glycemic Index (GI) is categorized as:

0-55   *Low GI*

56-69   *Medium GI*

70-above   *High GI*

b. fill half of your plate with varieties of veggies, most especially leafy greens, cruciferous vegetables, and non-starchy varieties.

c. Brown rice, quinoa, oats, and whole-wheat bread are examples of whole grains that are excellent for the body and can be substituted for refined grains.

d. Choose foods high in lean protein, such as tofu, beans, lentils, chicken, and fish.

e. Consume foods high in monounsaturated and polyunsaturated fats, such as avocados, nuts, seeds, and olive oil.

> If you want to manage your blood sugar levels effectively, you need to be mindful of the quantity of food you consume to avoid overeating. To determine the right portion sizes, use measuring cups, a kitchen scale, or your hands as visual indicators.

> Even though carbs are a vital component of a balanced diet, you must control your carbohydrate intake. Go for whole grains, fruits, and vegetables because they contain low-GI carbs. Plus, they break down sugar into the body gradually. You can combine carbs with fiber and protein to help your body reduce the absorption of blood sugar even more.

> Time your meals correctly to avoid energy dumps and to help normalize your blood sugar levels. You can eat three main meals and two to three snacks throughout the day, you can spread out these meals every three to four hours.

> Adjust your food plan to reflect your cultural background and personal taste preferences. Select

dishes and ingredients that suit your dietary customs and that you appreciate.

➢ Be creative with your dishes, don't give room for bland and uninteresting foods because of your prediabetes status. Rather, keep your meals interesting and fun, try out new recipes, play around with flavor combinations, and learn healthy cooking methods.

Do not forget that developing a healthy meal plan for someone with prediabetes is a continuous effort. As you discover new things about your body and what it demands, please take it easy, be flexible, and be open to changes. Always remember that you can gain the health goals and general well-being you desire with dedication and consistency.

"don't let minor setbacks discourage you. Keep moving forward, one healthy choice at a time."

NOTE

CHAPTER 3: DELICIOUS AND NUTRITIOUS RECIPES

Let's start with the vegetables. They are known to have abundance of vitamins and minerals that keep your body functioning properly, they act as the protectors of our health. See them your dependable soldiers who are available to help you at all times.

And then there are fruits, they are packed with lots of nutrients, taste, and they are a great source of fiber and antioxidants. Every time you bite into one, it's like giving your body a virtual high five.

Whole grains are another nutrient-rich food you should not overlook because they provide a stable base for your meals. They fill you up and supply you with energy. They are your dependable friend that has your back no matter what.

Start a 90-day journey with this delicious and nourishing food plan to fuel your body and control prediabetes. All recipes listed below are tested and trusted as they are what I used to regulate by blood sugar levels and promote overall well-being. You can fix the recipes to your taste.

Week 1	Breakfast	Lunch	Dinner	Snack
Monday	Oatmeal prepared from Creamy Berry topped with nuts and seeds	Grilled Chicken with Mixed greens, and light vinaigrette dressing	Roasted Vegetables serve with Baked Salmon	Apple cut and coated almond butter
Tuesday	Pancakes cooked from whole-wheat with fresh berries and a sprinkling of maple syrup	Quinoa Salad with chickpeas, cucumbers, red onion, and a lemon-tahini dressing	Turkey Meatballs with whole-wheat spaghetti and a side of steamed veggies	Carrot sticks with hummus
Wednesday	Scrambled eggs with spinach and feta cheese over whole-grain bread	Lentil Soup with a side salad and whole-grain crackers	Grilled Tofu with stir-fried veggies (bell peppers, onions, snow peas) and brown rice	Greek yogurt with a handful of berries and a sprinkle of honey

Thursday	Overnight Oats garnished with almond milk, chia seeds, and bananas	Veggie Wrap with whole-wheat tortillas, hummus, cucumber, tomato, and sprouts	Baked Salmon with Lemon and Herbs	Greek Yogurt Parfait
Friday	Smoothie prepared with almond milk, spinach, banana, and a scoop of protein powder	Tuna Salad Sandwich on whole-grain bread with lettuce, tomato, and avocado	Chicken Stir-fry with brown rice, broccoli, and a light soy sauce-based sauce	Rice cakes with sliced avocado and a sprinkling of black pepper
Saturday	Breakfast Burrito Bowl with scrambled eggs, black beans, salsa, and a dollop of Greek yogurt	Leftover Chicken Stir-fry with a side salad	Vegetaria n Chili with kidney beans, black beans, corn, tomatoes, and a dusting of spices	A bunch of grapes and a little slice of dark chocolate

Sunday	Whole-wheat waffles with fresh berries and a sprinkle of maple syrup	Black Bean Soup with a serving of whole-grain crackers	Grilled Shrimp Skewers with roasted zucchini and bell peppers	Cottage cheese with a sliced peach

Week 2

Monday	Avocado bread with mashed avocado, sliced tomato, and a sprinkling of hemp seeds over whole-grain bread	Salad Niçoise with mixed greens, tuna, hard-boiled eggs, olives, cherry tomatoes, and a mild vinaigrette	Baked Chicken Tenders with roasted Brussels sprouts and quinoa	Sliced banana served with rice cakes and peanut butter
Tuesday	Smoothie prepared with almond milk, mixed berries,	Leftover Vegetarian Chili with a side salad	Vegetarian Stuffed Peppers with quinoa, black beans,	A handful of almonds and dried cranberries

	and a scoop of collagen powder		corn, and a variety of spices	
Wednesday	Breakfast Frittata with spinach, mushrooms, and a sprinkling of cheese	Salad with grilled chicken, mixed greens, avocado, cherry tomatoes, and a mild vinaigrette	Whole Grain Pasta with Tomato and Basil	Greek yogurt with a handful of berries and a sprinkle of honey
Thursday	Overnight Oats with chia seeds, almond milk, sliced banana, and a sprinkling of cinnamon	Veggie Wrap with whole-wheat tortillas, hummus, cucumber, tomato, and sprouts	Chicken Stir-fry with brown rice, broccoli, and a light soy sauce-based sauce	A handful of mixed nuts and dry fruits
Friday	Smoothie prepared with almond milk, spinach, banana,	Tuna Salad Sandwich on whole-grain bread with lettuce,	Chicken and Vegetable Skewers	Rice cakes with sliced avocado and a sprinkling

	and a scoop of protein powder	tomato, and avocado		of black pepper
Saturday	Breakfast Burrito Bowl with scrambled eggs, black beans, salsa, and a dollop of Greek yogurt	Leftover Chicken Stir-fry with a side salad	Vegetarian Chili with kidney beans, black beans, corn, tomatoes, and a dusting of spices	A bunch of grapes and a little slice of dark chocolate
Sunday	Whole-wheat waffles with fresh berries and a sprinkle of maple syrup	Black Bean Soup with a serving of whole-grain crackers	Grilled Shrimp Skewers with roasted zucchini and bell peppers	Cottage cheese with a sliced peach
Week 3				
Monday	Avocado bread with mashed avocado, sliced	Salad Niçoise with mixed greens, tuna, hard-	Baked Chicken Tenders with roasted	Fruits mixed with Nuts Smoothie Bowl

	tomato, and a sprinkling of hemp seeds over whole-grain bread	boiled eggs, olives, cherry tomatoes, and a mild vinaigrette	Brussels sprouts and quinoa	
Tuesday	Smoothie prepared with almond milk, mixed berries, and a scoop of collagen powder	Leftover Vegetarian Chili with a side salad	Vegetaria n Stuffed Peppers with quinoa, black beans, corn, and a variety of spices	A handful of almonds and dried cranberrie s
Wednesday	Breakfast Frittata with spinach, mushroom s, and a sprinkling of cheese	Salad with grilled chicken, mixed greens, avocado, cherry tomatoes, and a mild vinaigrette	Baked Cod with Lemon and Herbs	Greek yogurt with a handful of berries and a sprinkle of honey
Thursday	Overnight Oats with chia seeds,	Veggie Wrap with whole-	Chicken Stir-fry with	A handful of mixed

	almond milk, sliced banana, and a sprinkling of cinnamon	wheat tortillas, hummus, cucumber, tomato, and sprouts	brown rice, broccoli, and a light soy sauce-based sauce	nuts and dry fruits
Friday	Smoothie prepared with almond milk, spinach, banana, and a scoop of protein powder	Tuna Salad Sandwich on whole-grain bread with lettuce, tomato, and avocado	Greek Chicken Salad	Rice cakes with sliced avocado and a sprinkling of black pepper
Saturday	Breakfast Burrito Bowl with scrambled eggs, black beans, salsa, and a dollop of Greek yogurt	Leftover Chicken Stir-fry with a side salad	Vegetarian Chili with kidney beans, black beans, corn, tomatoes, and a dusting of spices	A bunch of grapes and a little slice of dark chocolate

Sunday	Whole-wheat waffles with fresh berries and a sprinkle of maple syrup	Black Bean Soup with a serving of whole-grain crackers	Grilled Shrimp Skewers with roasted zucchini and bell peppers	Cottage cheese with a sliced peach
Week 4				
Monday	Avocado bread with mashed avocado, sliced tomato, and a sprinkling of hemp seeds over whole-grain bread	Salad Niçoise with mixed greens, tuna, hard-boiled eggs, olives, cherry tomatoes, and a mild vinaigrette	Baked Chicken Tenders with roasted Brussels sprouts and quinoa	Peanut Butter with Banana Smoothie
Tuesday	Smoothie prepared with almond milk, mixed berries, and a scoop of	Leftover Vegetarian Chili with a side salad	Vegetaria n Stuffed Peppers with quinoa, black beans, corn, and	A handful of almonds and dried cranberrie s

	collagen powder		a variety of spices
Wednesday	Breakfast Frittata with spinach, mushrooms, and a sprinkling of cheese	Salad with grilled chicken, mixed greens, avocado, cherry tomatoes, and a mild vinaigrette	Turkey and Veggie Lettuce Wraps	Greek yogurt with a handful of berries and a sprinkle of honey
Thursday	Overnight Oats with chia seeds, almond milk, sliced banana, and a sprinkling of cinnamon	Veggie Wrap with whole-wheat tortillas, hummus, cucumber, tomato, and sprouts	Chicken Stir-fry with brown rice, broccoli, and a light soy sauce-based sauce	A handful of mixed nuts and dry fruits
Friday	Smoothie prepared with almond milk, spinach, banana, and a scoop of	Tuna Salad Sandwich on whole-grain bread with lettuce, tomato, and avocado	Roasted sweet potatoes with grilled cod and asparagus	Rice cakes with sliced avocado and a sprinkling of black pepper

	protein powder			
Saturday	Breakfast Burrito Bowl with scrambled eggs, black beans, salsa, and a dollop of Greek yogurt	Leftover Chicken Stir-fry with a side salad	Vegetarian Chili with kidney beans, black beans, corn, tomatoes, and a dusting of spices	A bunch of grapes and a little slice of dark chocolate
Sunday	Whole-wheat waffles with fresh berries and a sprinkle of maple syrup	Black Bean Soup with a serving of whole-grain crackers	Grilled Shrimp Skewers with roasted zucchini and bell peppers	Cottage cheese with a sliced peach
Week 5				
Monday	Avocado bread with mashed avocado, sliced tomato, and a	Salad Niçoise with mixed greens, tuna, hard-boiled eggs,	Baked Chicken Tenders with roasted Brussels sprouts	Almond and Berry Salad

	sprinkling of hemp seeds over whole-grain bread	olives, cherry tomatoes, and a mild vinaigrette	and quinoa
Tuesday	Smoothie prepared with almond milk, mixed berries, and a scoop of collagen powder	Leftover Vegetarian Chili with a side salad	Vegetarian Stuffed Peppers with quinoa, black beans, corn, and a variety of spices	A handful of almonds and dried cranberries
Wednesday	Breakfast Frittata with spinach, mushrooms, and a sprinkling of cheese	Salad with grilled chicken, mixed greens, avocado, cherry tomatoes, and a mild vinaigrette	Grilled Veggie and Hummus Pizza	Broccoli and baby carrots with yoghurt dip
Thursday	Overnight Oats with chia seeds, almond milk,	Veggie Wrap with whole-wheat tortillas,	Chicken Stir-fry with brown rice,	A handful of mixed nuts and dry fruits

	sliced banana, and a sprinkling of cinnamon	hummus, cucumber, tomato, and sprouts	broccoli, and a light soy sauce-based sauce	
Friday	Smoothie prepared with almond milk, spinach, banana, and a scoop of protein powder	Tuna Salad Sandwich on whole-grain bread with lettuce, tomato, and avocado	Sweet Potato and Black Bean Enchiladas	Rice cakes with sliced avocado and a sprinkling of black pepper
Saturday	Breakfast Burrito Bowl with scrambled eggs, black beans, salsa, and a dollop of Greek yogurt	Leftover Chicken Stir-fry with a side salad	Vegetarian Chili with kidney beans, black beans	
Sunday	Whole-wheat waffles with fresh	Black Bean Soup with a serving of whole-	Grilled Shrimp Skewers with	Cottage cheese with a

berries and a sprinkle of maple syrup	grain crackers	roasted zucchini and bell peppers	sliced peach

Week 6

Monday

Avocado bread with mashed avocado, sliced tomato, and a sprinkling of hemp seeds over whole-grain bread	Salad Niçoise with mixed greens, tuna, hard-boiled eggs, olives, cherry tomatoes, and a mild vinaigrette	Baked Chicken Tenders with roasted Brussels sprouts and quinoa	Berry with Spinach Smoothie Bowl

Tuesday

Smoothie prepared with almond milk, mixed berries, and a scoop of collagen powder	Leftover Vegetarian Chili with a side salad	Vegetarian Stuffed Peppers with quinoa, black beans, corn, and a variety of spices	A handful of almonds and dried cranberries

	Breakfast	Lunch	Dinner	Snack
Wednesday	Breakfast Frittata with spinach, mushrooms, and a sprinkling of cheese	Salad with grilled chicken, mixed greens, avocado, cherry tomatoes, and a mild vinaigrette	Mango Avocado Quinoa Bowl	Greek yogurt with a handful of berries and a sprinkle of honey
Thursday	Overnight Oats with chia seeds, almond milk, sliced banana, and a sprinkling of cinnamon	Veggie Wrap with whole-wheat tortillas, hummus, cucumber, tomato, and sprouts	Chicken Stir-fry with brown rice, broccoli, and a light soy sauce-based sauce	A handful of mixed nuts and dry fruits
Friday	Smoothie prepared with almond milk, spinach, banana, and a scoop of protein powder	Tuna Salad Sandwich on whole-grain bread with lettuce, tomato, and avocado	Turkey and Avocado Wrap	Rice cakes with sliced avocado and a sprinkling of black pepper

Saturday	Breakfast Burrito Bowl with scrambled eggs, black beans, salsa, and a dollop of Greek yogurt	Leftover Chicken Stir-fry with a side salad	Vegetaria n Chili with kidney beans, black beans, corn, tomatoes, and a dusting of spices	A bunch of grapes and a little slice of dark chocolate
Sunday	Whole-wheat waffles with fresh berries and a sprinkle of maple syrup	Black Bean Soup with a serving of whole-grain crackers	Grilled Shrimp Skewers with roasted zucchini and bell peppers	Cottage cheese with a sliced peach
Week 7				
Monday	Avocado bread with mashed avocado, sliced tomato, and a sprinkling of hemp seeds over	Salad Niçoise with mixed greens, tuna, hard-boiled eggs, olives, cherry tomatoes,	Baked Chicken Tenders with roasted Brussels sprouts and quinoa	Mango and Coconut Chia Parfait

	whole-grain bread	and a mild vinaigrette		
Tuesday	Smoothie prepared with almond milk, mixed berries, and a scoop of collagen powder	Leftover Vegetarian Chili with a side salad	Vegetarian Stuffed Peppers with quinoa, black beans, corn, and a variety of spices	A handful of almonds and dried cranberries
Wednesday	Breakfast Frittata with spinach, mushrooms, and a sprinkling of cheese	Salad with grilled chicken, mixed greens, avocado, cherry tomatoes, and a mild vinaigrette	Roasted Sweet Potatoes with grilled salmon and Kale	Greek yogurt with a handful of berries and a sprinkle of honey
Thursday	Overnight Oats with chia seeds, almond milk, sliced banana, and a	Veggie Wrap with whole-wheat tortillas, hummus, cucumber,	Chicken Stir-fry with brown rice, broccoli, and a light soy sauce-	A handful of mixed nuts and dry fruits

	sprinkling of cinnamon	tomato, and sprouts	based sauce	
Friday	Smoothie prepared with almond milk, spinach, banana, and a scoop of protein powder	Tuna Salad Sandwich on whole-grain bread with lettuce, tomato, and avocado	Healthy Cauliflower and Chickpea Tacos	Rice cakes with sliced avocado and a sprinkling of black pepper
Saturday	Breakfast Burrito Bowl with scrambled eggs, black beans, salsa, and a dollop of Greek yogurt	Leftover Chicken Stir-fry with a side salad	Vegetarian Chili with kidney beans, black beans, corn, tomatoes, and a dusting of spices	Strawberry and Banana Chia Pudding
Sunday	Whole-wheat waffles with fresh berries and a	Black Bean Soup with a serving of whole-grain crackers	Grilled Shrimp Skewers with roasted zucchini	Banana, apples with almond milk

sprinkle of maple syrup		and bell peppers	smoothie bowl

Week 8				
Monday	Avocado bread with mashed avocado, sliced tomato, and a sprinkling of hemp seeds over whole-grain bread	Salad Niçoise with mixed greens, tuna, hard-boiled eggs, olives, cherry tomatoes, and a mild vinaigrette	Baked Chicken Tenders with roasted Brussels sprouts and quinoa	Peanut butter and banana slices with rice cake
Tuesday	Smoothie prepared with almond milk, mixed berries, and a scoop of collagen powder	Leftover Vegetarian Chili with a side salad	Vegetarian Stuffed Peppers with quinoa, black beans, corn, and a variety of spices	A handful of almonds and dried cranberries
Wednesday	Breakfast Frittata with	Salad with grilled chicken,	Spinach and Feta Omelette	Greek yogurt with a

	spinach, mushrooms, and a sprinkling of cheese	mixed greens, avocado, cherry tomatoes, and a mild vinaigrette		handful of berries and a sprinkle of honey
Thursday	Overnight Oats with chia seeds, almond milk, sliced banana, and a sprinkling of cinnamon	Veggie Wrap with whole-wheat tortillas, hummus, cucumber, tomato, and sprouts	Chicken Stir-fry with brown rice, broccoli, and a light soy sauce-based sauce	A handful of mixed nuts and dry fruits
Friday	Smoothie prepared with almond milk, spinach, banana, and a scoop of protein powder	Tuna Salad Sandwich on whole-grain bread with lettuce, tomato, and avocado	Veggie Frittata	Rice cakes with sliced avocado and a sprinkling of black pepper Saturday
Saturday	Breakfast Burrito Bowl with	Leftover Chicken Stir-fry	Vegetarian Chili with	A bunch of grapes and a little

	scrambled eggs, black beans, salsa, and a dollop of Greek yogurt	with a side salad	kidney beans, black beans, corn, tomatoes, and a dusting of spices	slice of dark chocolate
Sunday	Whole-wheat waffles with fresh berries and a sprinkle of maple syrup	Black Bean Soup with a serving of whole-grain crackers	Grilled Shrimp Skewers with roasted zucchini and bell peppers	Cottage cheese with a sliced peach
Week 9				
Monday	Avocado bread with mashed avocado, sliced tomato, and a sprinkling of hemp seeds over whole-grain bread	Salad Niçoise with mixed greens, tuna, hard-boiled eggs, olives, cherry tomatoes, and a mild vinaigrette	Baked Chicken Tenders with roasted Brussels sprouts and quinoa	Spinach, cucumber, banana and almond milk smoothie

Tuesday	Smoothie prepared with almond milk, mixed berries, and a scoop of collagen powder	Leftover Vegetarian Chili with a side salad	Vegetarian Stuffed Peppers with quinoa, black beans, corn, and a variety of spices	A handful of almonds and dried cranberries
Wednesday	Breakfast Frittata with spinach, mushrooms, and a sprinkling of cheese	Salad with grilled chicken, mixed greens, avocado, cherry tomatoes, and a mild vinaigrette	Baked Eggplant Parmesan	Greek yogurt with a handful of berries and a sprinkle of honey
Thursday	Overnight Oats with chia seeds, almond milk, sliced banana, and a sprinkling of cinnamon	Veggie Wrap with whole-wheat tortillas, hummus, cucumber, tomato, and sprouts	Chicken Stir-fry with brown rice, broccoli, and a light soy sauce-based sauce	A handful of mixed nuts and dry fruits

Friday	Smoothie prepared with almond milk, spinach, banana, and a scoop of protein powder	Tuna Salad Sandwich on whole-grain bread with lettuce, tomato, and avocado	Butternut Squash and Chickpea Curry	Rice cakes with sliced avocado and a sprinkling of black pepper
Saturday	Breakfast Burrito Bowl with scrambled eggs, black beans, salsa, and a dollop of Greek yogurt	Leftover Chicken Stir-fry with a side salad	Vegetarian Chili with kidney beans, black beans, corn, tomatoes, and a dusting of spices	A bunch of grapes and a little slice of dark chocolate
Sunday	Whole-wheat waffles with fresh berries and a sprinkle of maple syrup	Black Bean Soup with a serving of whole-grain crackers	Grilled Shrimp Skewers with roasted zucchini and bell peppers	Cottage cheese with a sliced peach

Week 10

Monday	Avocado bread with mashed avocado, sliced tomato, and a sprinkling of hemp seeds over whole-grain bread	Salad Niçoise with mixed greens, tuna, hard-boiled eggs, olives, cherry tomatoes, and a mild vinaigrette	Baked Chicken Tenders with roasted Brussels sprouts and quinoa	A fits full of mixed nuts
Tuesday	Smoothie prepared with almond milk, mixed berries, and a scoop of collagen powder	Leftover Vegetarian Chili with a side salad	Vegetarian Stuffed Peppers with quinoa, black beans, corn, and a variety of spices	A handful of almonds and dried cranberries
Wednesday	Breakfast Frittata with spinach, mushrooms, and a	Salad with grilled chicken, mixed greens, avocado, cherry	Baked Salmon with steamed colorful veggies	Greek yogurt with a handful of berries and a

	sprinkling of cheese	tomatoes, and a mild vinaigrette		sprinkle of honey
Thursday	Overnight Oats with chia seeds, almond milk, sliced banana, and a sprinkling of cinnamon	Veggie Wrap with whole-wheat tortillas, hummus, cucumber, tomato, and sprouts	Chicken Stir-fry with brown rice, broccoli, and a light soy sauce-based sauce	A handful of mixed nuts and dry fruits
Friday	Smoothie prepared with almond milk, spinach, banana, and a scoop of protein powder	Tuna Salad Sandwich on whole-grain bread with lettuce, tomato, and avocado	Baked sweet potatoes with grilled cod and broccoli	Rice cakes with sliced avocado and a sprinkling of black pepper
Saturday	Breakfast Burrito Bowl with scrambled eggs, black beans,	Leftover Chicken Stir-fry with a side salad	Vegetarian Chili with kidney beans, black beans,	A bunch of grapes and a little slice of dark chocolate

	salsa, and a dollop of Greek yogurt		corn, tomatoes, and a dusting of spices	
Sunday	Whole-wheat waffles with fresh berries and a sprinkle of maple syrup	Black Bean Soup with a serving of whole-grain crackers	Grilled Shrimp Skewers with roasted zucchini and bell peppers	Cottage cheese with a sliced peach
Week 11				
Monday	Avocado bread with mashed avocado, sliced tomato, and a sprinkling of hemp seeds over whole-grain bread	Salad Niçoise with mixed greens, tuna, hard-boiled eggs, olives, cherry tomatoes, and a mild vinaigrette	Baked Chicken Tenders with roasted Brussels sprouts and quinoa	Rice cakes with peanut butter and sliced banana
Tuesday	Smoothie prepared with	Leftover Vegetarian	Vegetarian Stuffed Peppers	A handful of almonds

	almond milk, mixed berries, and a scoop of collagen powder	Chili with a side salad	with quinoa, black beans, corn, and a variety of spices	and dried cranberries
Wednesday	Breakfast Frittata with spinach, mushrooms, and a sprinkling of cheese	Salad with grilled chicken, mixed greens, avocado, cherry tomatoes, and a mild vinaigrette	Baked Salmon with Roasted Sweet Potatoes and Kale	Greek yogurt with a handful of berries and a sprinkle of honey
Thursday	Overnight Oats with chia seeds, almond milk, sliced banana, and a sprinkling of cinnamon	Veggie Wrap with whole-wheat tortillas, hummus, cucumber, tomato, and sprouts	Chicken Stir-fry with brown rice, broccoli, and a light soy sauce-based sauce	A handful of mixed nuts and dry fruits
Friday	Smoothie prepared with	Tuna Salad Sandwich on whole-	Baked Cod with roasted	Rice cakes with sliced

	almond milk, spinach, banana, and a scoop of protein powder	grain bread with lettuce, tomato, and avocado	sweet potatoes and asparagus	avocado and a sprinkling of black pepper
Saturday	Whole-wheat pancakes with fresh berries and a sprinkle of maple syrup	Quinoa Salad with chickpeas, cucumbers, red onion, and a lemon-tahini dressing	Turkey Meatballs with whole-wheat spaghetti and a side of steamed veggies	
Sunday	Breakfast Frittata with spinach, mushrooms, and a sprinkling of cheese	Salad with grilled chicken, mixed greens, avocado, cherry tomatoes, and a mild vinaigrette	Baked Sweet Potatoes with grilled salmon and Kale	Greek yogurt with a handful of berries and a sprinkle of honey
Week 12				
Monday	Avocado bread with	Salad Niçoise	Baked Chicken	Banana and apple

	mashed avocado, sliced tomato, and a sprinkling of hemp seeds over whole-grain bread	with mixed greens, tuna, hard-boiled eggs, olives, cherry tomatoes, and a mild vinaigrette	Tenders with roasted Brussels sprouts and quinoa	slices coated in peanut butter
Tuesday	Scrambled eggs with spinach and feta cheese over whole-grain bread	Lentil Soup with a side salad and whole-grain crackers	Grilled Tofu with stir-fried veggies (bell peppers, onions, snow peas) and brown rice	Greek yogurt with a handful of berries and a sprinkle of honey

Please note that this is just a sample meal plan, and you may need to adjust the recipes to your preference.

NOTE

_____

_____

_____

_____

_____

_____

_____

_____

_____

_____

_____

_____

_____

_____

_____

_____

_____

NOTE

NOTE

_____

_____

_____

_____

_____

_____

_____

_____

_____

_____

_____

_____

_____

_____

_____

CHAPTER 4: PORTION CONTROL

Every food group on your plate is important and perform a unique function in the progress of your health. However, having too little size of vegetables or too much of carbohydrate on the plate can create an imbalance. This is why portion control is key when plating your meal.

Portion control simply means eating the right amount of each food groups. The purpose of measuring foods when plating is not to prevent you from enjoying your favorite foods, but to guide you in eating the proper quantity.

You need to know that portion sizes help to balance your meal. Proteins, carbohydrates, and vegetables all play a part in your diet, and when they all come together, it boosts your health.

MY TABLE

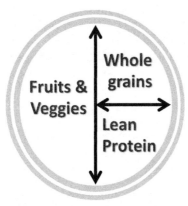

The following is the recommended serving size of food:

- *Vegetables:* Get a plate and cover half of it with vibrant vegetables. Yes, mix different colors! These are your go-to vegetables, so eat a lot of them.

- *Proteins:* select your choice of protein, be it tofu, fish, poultry, or beans. Try to get a quantity about the size of your hand or quarter of your plate

- *Carbohydrates:* fill the quarter of your dish with whole grains or potatoes. It performs a function in your diet.

- *Don't overlook the fats!* Healthy fats, such as olive oil, and avocado are excellent choice as they enhance flavor and keep your meal interesting. You can include about a thumb size in your meal.

- *Extras:* you can garnish your dish with little quantity of almonds or a dollop of yogurt if space permits. These are the unexpected components that set your dish apart.

Do not forget that balance is all that matter and not perfection. Use your hand as a guide when plating your meal, and trust your gut. Ensure you enjoy the sumptuous dish you've made.

NOTE

_____

_____

_____

_____

_____

_____

_____

_____

_____

_____

_____

_____

_____

_____

_____

NOTE

CHAPTER 5: THE GROCERY GUIDE

To make healthy meals, you need a healthy shopping list. This list guides you in selecting the right foods into your shopping basket. But first, let's discuss the grocery guide:

1. Go with a grocery list. When you do this, it helps you stay focused and resist impulsive purchases. Make a list of the vegetables, fruits, grains, and proteins you'll need for the coming week.

2. focus your attention on the store's perimeter. This is where you will get fresh fruit, meats, and dairy products—real, and whole foods.

3. colors boost the mood. So, select colorful fresh produce like fruits and vegetables into your cart.

4. Read labels (but don't get too technical!). check the label on the item to see the nutritional facts. Also, to know if it is organic and unprocessed. Do not forget that organic and unprocessed foods are the best option.

5. Never go shopping on empty stomach. Make sure to snack on something before you leave the house to avoid being allured by sugary sweets.

Vegetables:

Broccoli

Spinach

Kale

Brussels sprouts

Cauliflower

Bell peppers (various colors)

Zucchini

Cucumbers

Tomatoes

Carrots

Fruits:

Berries (blueberries, strawberries, raspberries)

Apples

Pears

Oranges

Grapefruit (to be excepted by anyone who is on certain med.)

Kiwi

Cherries

Peaches

Plums

Grapes (to be excepted by anyone who is on certain med.)

Proteins:

Skinless chicken breast

Turkey

Salmon

Tofu

Eggs

Lentils

Chickpeas

Kidney beans

Black beans

Lean ground beef or turkey

Whole Grains:

Quinoa

Brown rice

Oats (steel-cut or rolled)

Whole wheat pasta

Barley

Farro

Bulgur

Whole grain bread

Whole grain tortillas

Buckwheat

Healthy Fats:

Avocado

Olive oil

Nuts (almonds, walnuts, pistachios)

Seeds (chia seeds, flaxseeds)

Nut butter (almond or peanut butter)

Fatty fish (mackerel, sardines)

Dairy or Dairy Alternatives:

Low-fat or skim milk

Greek yogurt (unsweetened)

Cheese (preferably low-fat)

Almond or soy milk (unsweetened)

Snacks:

Hummus

Raw veggies for snacking

Air-popped popcorn

Edamame

Greek yogurt with berries

Herbs and Spices:

Garlic

Ginger

Cinnamon

Turmeric

Fresh herbs (parsley, cilantro, basil)

Beverages:

Green tea (unsweetened)

Herbal tea (unsweetened)

Water with lemon or cucumber

Sparkling water (unsweetened)

Condiments:

Balsamic vinegar

Olive oil-based dressings

Mustard (Dijon or whole grain)

Salsa (low-sodium)

Low-sodium soy sauce

Tomato sauce (unsweetened)

Always look for natural, unadulterated meals and look out for added sugars on product labels. In order to support a balanced meal plan for prediabetes, this special grocery list focuses on fresh, whole foods that provide lots of nutrients.

NOTE

NOTE

_____

_____

_____

_____

_____

_____

_____

_____

_____

_____

_____

_____

_____

_____

_____

CHAPTER 6: MAKING IT SUSTAINABLE

I know that changing your diet might be difficult. This is why I have provided useful tactics to help you get beyond the challenges most beginners encounter. This book contains tips to help you with **proper planning**, and way to be motivated as you start the process.

1. Start small. Don't try to overhaul your entire diet overnight. Instead, make small, gradual changes that you can stick with over time.

2. Eat more of whole, unprocessed foods because they are high in fiber and minerals and can help control your sugar levels.

3. Always ensure you add protein to your dish. This is because it slows sugar absorption in the bloodstream.

4. Select good fats like nuts, seeds, avocados, and other healthy fats. They can all assist to increase insulin sensitivity.

5. Limit your intake of sugar-filled beverages. These beverages are a primary cause of diabetes and prediabetes. So, go for water, black coffee, or unsweetened tea instead.

6. Make cooking at home a priority. This will give you more control over the ingredients in your meals.

7. Plan your meals ahead of time. This will help you to make healthy choices when you're short on time.

8. Don't be afraid to try out new recipes, there are endless possibilities when it comes to healthy cooking. Try new recipes and find what you enjoy.

9. Involve your family in meal planning and cooking. This will help everyone to eat healthier.

10. Be patient. It takes time to make lasting changes to your diet. Take it easy on with yourself nd never give up.

"never forget, your health is worth it.

invest in your health today, and start

living your best life."

CHAPTER 7: SUCCESS STORIES AND RESOURCES

I remember when I was newly diagnosed with prediabetes. In an attempt to overcome my worries, I joined a social media prediabetes community. Then, I stumbled on stories shared by people. The good, the not-so-good, and everything in between. Based on all I read, it was glaring that many people didn't pay much attention to the signs of prediabetes until it knocked on their door just like mine.

This is not intended to frighten you; rather, to remind you that sometimes we only need a reminder to get started on changing things.

Here are top two stories that struck my attention on the platform, and gave me hope during my fight against prediabetes.

"Hey, I'm John Crawford, a 52-year-old man. I was diagnosed with prediabetes. Thanks to my family and my doctor, I was introduced to a pre-diabetes meal plan and exercising which changed my health completely. I implemented everything on the meal plan and made little dietary adjustments, including choosing healthy grains over processed grains and eating lots of fruits and vegetables.

Within the first 4months of using the meal plan, I was able to lose ten pounds. My blood sugar levels returned to normal after a year".

David Rodrigez, a 60-year-old man, with prediabetes. He was committed to altering his way of living in order to prevent the onset of diabetes. He began going for thirty-minute walks most days of the week. In addition, he altered his diet, cutting back on processed foods and sweets. His blood sugar levels returned to normal within six months.

These are few of the people who have effectively reversed prediabetes. You can too, with the correct lifestyle adjustments.

"prediabetes is a chance for you to make positive changes and create a healthier lifestyle."

NOTE

_____

_____

_____

_____

_____

_____

_____

_____

_____

_____

_____

_____

_____

_____

_____

NOTE

_____
_____
_____
_____
_____
_____
_____
_____
_____
_____
_____
_____
_____
_____
_____
_____

CHAPTER 8: BEYOND THE PLATE

Based on all you learned from chapters before this, you already know that diet is very important in reversing prediabetes. However, there are other factors that can help speed up the process. These factors are consistent exercise, stress reduction, and getting enough sleep.

In this section, I will go into the emotional aspects of controlling prediabetes. Here, you will learn the various emotions that comes with prediabetes and how to overcome them. Trust me, you're not alone.

1. Having prediabetes can cause roller-coaster of emotions. This is absolutely normal and fine. It may feel like a bit of a struggle some days, and other days you can feel inspired and on top of the world. This is understandable.

2. When you take a bold step of actualizing a dream. No matter how little you do, you deserve to celebrate yourself because every step is a victory. Celebrate yourself when you snack on healthy foods or when you take an early morning stroll. These little steps build up positive results and encourages you to do more.

3. There are days you may feel emotionally down, frustrated or nervous. It is normal to feel this way. It is not a sign of failure. This only means you are human. So don't beat yourself down. Rather, allow those emotions, and then encourage yourself not to give up. Let the health goals you want to achieve motivate you to keep pushing.

4. Think of your friends and family as your support squad. Share your journey with them. Let them cheer you on and be there for you when you need a boost. You're not alone in this.

5. Remember, this is your life and your health. Every choice you make for your health is a step towards a healthier, happier you. Always tell yourself that you are in control, and you're doing something amazing for yourself.

"you have the power to correct your health. Take control now, and change the narrative.

NOTE

_____

_____

_____

_____

_____

_____

_____

_____

_____

_____

_____

_____

_____

_____

_____

_____

NOTE

_____
_____
_____
_____
_____
_____
_____
_____
_____
_____
_____
_____
_____
_____
_____
_____

CONCLUSION: EMBRACING YOUR JOURNEY

Now that we are at the final lap of this book, take a minute to reflect on all those small wins - the days you went for a walk, the colorful salads you selected, and the times you go for healthy fruit instead of a sweet snack. They are your victories, and you deserve to be celebrated.

Do not forget that you are not alone in this. You have people who love and support your health decisions. Your family and friends are there cheering you on. You can always rely on them when necessary, share your joy with them when you can, and allow their encouragement to uplift you.

Every action you have made, and every decision you have taken either big or small during this process, is a step closer to being a better version of yourself. You deserve to pat yourself on the back for your accomplishments. You're phenomenal!

The power to rewrite your story is in your hands my friend. You are the one with the pen, and prediabetes is only but a chapter. To achieve that health goal, you desire so much, continue to make the decisions that uplift your mood, promote your health, and give you pride.

Don't forget that it is not over yet. The process continues. However, you have the right knowledge, and support you need to make positive changes to your health.

As we get to the end of this chapter, remember to love and cherish who you are. You've accepted both the mental and physical aspects of managing prediabetes. You're strong, resilient, and moving in the direction of a better, happier version of yourself. To your adventure, your successes, and the incredible chapters that lies ahead, I say

cheers!

REFERENCE

The American Diabetes Association: https://diabetes.org/about-diabetes/prediabetes

The Centers for Disease Control and Prevention: https://www.cdc.gov/chronicdisease/resources/publications/factsheets/diabetes-prediabetes.htm

The National Institute of Diabetes and Digestive and Kidney Diseases: https://www.ncbi.nlm.nih.gov/books/NBK459332/

The Prediabetes Coalition: https://doihaveprediabetes.org/

Three-Month Prediabetes Workout Plan:

This program combines strength and aerobic training to help:

a. Maintain weight

b. Improve blood sugar regulation

c. And increase energy

Remember, listen to your body and adjust intensity accordingly.

First Month:

Focus: Learning correct form and increasing foundational fitness.

Cardio:

Engage in 30 minutes' brisk walk, for at least five days a week. You can increase duration by 5 minutes for each week.

Swimming:

Engage yourself in swimming twice a week, for 20 minutes. You can focus on different strokes.

Strength Training:

2-3 days a week of full-body exercise interspersed with rest days. 2 sets of 10-12 repetitions with light weights or bodyweight.

DAYS	FOR 30 MINUTES	FOR 20 MINUTES
MONDAY	Brisk walk (Aim for 10,000 steps)	Rest
TUESDAY	Full-body exercise (2 sets of 10-12 repetitions of squats and lunges)	Swimming (freestyle)
WEDNESDAY	Brisk walk (Aim for 10,000 steps)	Rest
THURSDAY	Full-body exercise (2 sets of 10-12 repetitions of push-ups and rows)	Swimming (backstroke)
FRIDAY	Brisk walk (Aim for 10,000 steps)	Rest
SATURDAY	Brisk walk	Full-body exercise (2

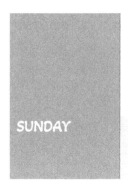	(Aim for 10,000 steps)	sets of 10-12 repetitions of rows and planks)
SUNDAY	Brisk walk (Aim for 10,000 steps)	Rest

Second Month:

Focus: Increasing intensity and adding new exercises.

Cardio:

Interval training: Alternate between walking and jogging/running for 35 minutes, 3 days/week.

Cycling:

35 minutes, 2-3 days/week. To enhance difficulty, change up the landscape.

Strength Training:

Split into two to three upper and lower body workout days each week, with rest days in between. three sets of light weighted repetitions (12–15 reps).

DAYS	FOR 35 MINUTES	FOR 30 MINUTES
MONDAY	Jogging	Cycling (increase landscape)
TUESDAY	Upper body exercise (3 sets of 12-15 repetitions of bicep curls and shoulder presses)	Rest
WEDNESDAY	Running	Cycling (increase landscape)
THURSDAY	upper body exercise (3 sets of 12-15 repetitions of dumbbell and triceps)	Rest
FRIDAY	Brisk walk (Aim for 11,000 steps)	Cycling (increase landscape)
SATURDAY	Lower body exercise (3 sets of 12-15 repetitions of	Rest

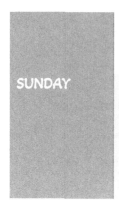		squats and calf raises)
SUNDAY	Rest	Lower body exercise (3 sets of 12-15 repetitions of deadlifts and lunges)

Third Month:

Focus: Adding new activities while keeping the intensity high.

Cardio:

High-Intensity Interval Training (HIIT): two to three days a week for 20 to 30 minutes. Combine intervals of rest (walking) with high-intensity exercise.

Dance fitness:

twice a week, for thirty minutes. Pick a dance style that you like.

Strength Training:

Two to three days a week, a full-body circuit with days off in between. 3 sets of moderate-to-heavy weight, 15-20 reps each.

Work out back-to-back with little to no break in between.

DAYS	FOR 20-30 MINUTES	FOR 30 MINUTES
MONDAY	Do jumping jacks and walking simultaneously	Salsa / Zumba dance
TUESDAY	Full-body exercise (3 sets of 15-20 repetitions of burpees to planks)	
WEDNESDAY	Do sprints and walking simultaneously	
THURSDAY	Full-body exercise (3 sets of 15-20 repetitions of push-ups to rows)	
FRIDAY	Do jumping jacks and walking simultaneously	Salsa / Zumba dance
SATURDAY	Full-body exercise (3 sets of 15-20 repetitions of squats to lunges)	

Salsa / Zumba
dance

Advantages of exercise for prediabetes

- Cardio boosts oxygen intake, helps burn calories, and raises insulin sensitivity, which makes it possible for your body to use glucose more effectively.
- Gaining muscle mass with strength training raises your metabolic rate and helps you burn more calories even while you're at rest. Moreover, stronger muscles enhance glucose absorption.
- HIIT: Increases insulin sensitivity and burns more calories faster than steady-state aerobic exercise.
- Being consistent matters a lot. The best strategy to control prediabetes and avoid type 2 diabetes is to exercise on a regular basis and maintain a healthy diet.

More Tips

- Spend five to ten minutes doing dynamic stretches and brief aerobics to warm up before every session.
- Afterward, do static stretches to decompress.
- Drink plenty of water throughout the day.
- Monitor your development to observe your gains and maintain motivation.
- Honor your accomplishments!

Before beginning any new fitness activity, especially if you have any health issues, speak with a healthcare provider.

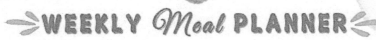

WEEKLY Meal PLANNER

Monday

Tuesday

Wednesday

Thursday

Friday

Saturday

Sunday

Shopping List:

_____
_____
_____
_____
_____
_____
_____
_____
_____
_____
_____
_____
_____
_____
_____
_____
_____
_____
_____

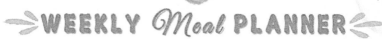

WEEKLY *Meal* PLANNER

Monday

Tuesday

Wednesday

Thursday

Friday

Saturday

Sunday

Shopping List:

_____
_____
_____
_____
_____
_____
_____
_____
_____
_____
_____
_____
_____
_____
_____
_____
_____
_____
_____

➤WEEKLY *Meal* PLANNER➤

Monday

Tuesday

Wednesday

Thursday

Friday

Saturday

Sunday

Shopping List:

_____
_____
_____
_____
_____
_____
_____
_____
_____
_____
_____
_____
_____
_____
_____
_____
_____
_____
_____
_____
_____

WEEKLY *Meal* PLANNER

Monday

Tuesday

Wednesday

Thursday

Friday

Saturday

Sunday

Shopping List:

WEEKLY Meal PLANNER

Monday

Tuesday

Wednesday

Thursday

Friday

Saturday

Sunday

Shopping List:

_____
_____
_____
_____
_____
_____
_____
_____
_____
_____
_____
_____
_____
_____
_____
_____
_____
_____
_____
_____

WEEKLY *Meal* PLANNER

Monday

Tuesday

Wednesday

Thursday

Friday

Saturday

Sunday

Shopping List:

_____
_____
_____
_____
_____
_____
_____
_____
_____
_____
_____
_____
_____
_____
_____
_____
_____
_____
_____
_____
_____
_____

WEEKLY Meal PLANNER

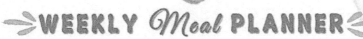

Monday	Shopping List:
Tuesday	_____
Wednesday	_____
Thursday	_____
Friday	_____
Saturday	_____
Sunday	_____

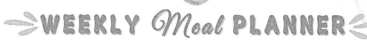

WEEKLY *Meal* PLANNER

Monday

Tuesday

Wednesday

Thursday

Friday

Saturday

Sunday

Shopping List:

_____
_____
_____
_____
_____
_____
_____
_____
_____
_____
_____
_____
_____
_____
_____
_____
_____
_____

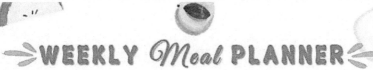

WEEKLY *Meal* PLANNER

Monday

Tuesday

Wednesday

Thursday

Friday

Saturday

Sunday

Shopping List:

_____
_____
_____
_____
_____
_____
_____
_____
_____
_____
_____
_____
_____
_____
_____
_____
_____
_____

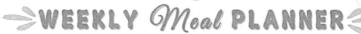

WEEKLY *Meal* PLANNER

Monday

Tuesday

Wednesday

Thursday

Friday

Saturday

Sunday

Shopping List:

_____
_____
_____
_____
_____
_____
_____
_____
_____
_____
_____
_____
_____
_____
_____
_____
_____
_____

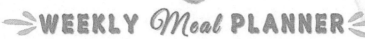

WEEKLY *Meal* PLANNER

| Monday | Shopping List: |

Monday

Tuesday

Wednesday

Thursday

Friday

Saturday

Sunday

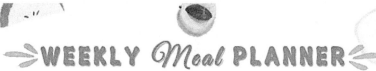

WEEKLY *Meal* PLANNER

Monday

Tuesday

Wednesday

Thursday

Friday

Saturday

Sunday

Shopping List:

_____
_____
_____
_____
_____
_____
_____
_____
_____
_____
_____
_____
_____
_____
_____
_____
_____
_____
_____
_____
_____

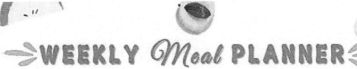

WEEKLY Meal PLANNER

Monday

Tuesday

Wednesday

Thursday

Friday

Saturday

Sunday

Shopping List:

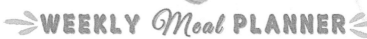

WEEKLY *Meal* PLANNER

Monday

Tuesday

Wednesday

Thursday

Friday

Saturday

Sunday

Shopping List:

_____

_____

_____

_____

_____

_____

_____

_____

_____

_____

_____

_____

_____

_____

_____

_____

_____

_____

WEEKLY *Meal* PLANNER

Monday

Tuesday

Wednesday

Thursday

Friday

Saturday

Sunday

Shopping List:

_____
_____
_____
_____
_____
_____
_____
_____
_____
_____
_____
_____
_____
_____
_____
_____
_____
_____
_____
_____
_____
_____
_____

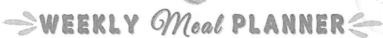

WEEKLY *Meal* PLANNER

Monday

Tuesday

Wednesday

Thursday

Friday

Saturday

Sunday

Shopping List:

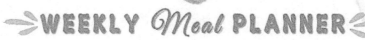

WEEKLY *Meal* PLANNER

Monday

Tuesday

Wednesday

Thursday

Friday

Saturday

Sunday

Shopping List:

_____
_____
_____
_____
_____
_____
_____
_____
_____
_____
_____
_____
_____
_____
_____
_____
_____
_____
_____
_____
_____

WEEKLY *Meal* PLANNER

Monday

Tuesday

Wednesday

Thursday

Friday

Saturday

Sunday

Shopping List:

_____
_____
_____
_____
_____
_____
_____
_____
_____
_____
_____
_____
_____
_____
_____
_____
_____
_____
_____
_____

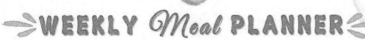

WEEKLY Meal PLANNER

Monday

Tuesday

Wednesday

Thursday

Friday

Saturday

Sunday

Shopping List:

_____
_____
_____
_____
_____
_____
_____
_____
_____
_____
_____
_____
_____
_____
_____
_____
_____
_____
_____

WEEKLY *Meal* PLANNER

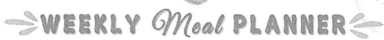

Monday

Tuesday

Wednesday

Thursday

Friday

Saturday

Sunday

Shopping List:

_____
_____
_____
_____
_____
_____
_____
_____
_____
_____
_____
_____
_____
_____
_____
_____
_____
_____
_____
_____
_____

WEEKLY *Meal* PLANNER

Monday

Tuesday

Wednesday

Thursday

Friday

Saturday

Sunday

Shopping List:

_____
_____
_____
_____
_____
_____
_____
_____
_____
_____
_____
_____
_____
_____
_____
_____
_____
_____
_____
_____
_____

WEEKLY *Meal* PLANNER

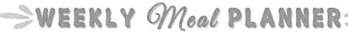

Monday

Tuesday

Wednesday

Thursday

Friday

Saturday

Sunday

Shopping List:

_____
_____
_____
_____
_____
_____
_____
_____
_____
_____
_____
_____
_____
_____
_____
_____
_____
_____
_____
_____
_____
_____
_____

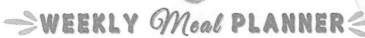

WEEKLY *Meal* PLANNER

Monday

Tuesday

Wednesday

Thursday

Friday

Saturday

Sunday

Shopping List:

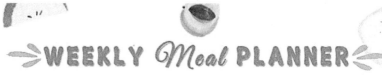

WEEKLY *Meal* PLANNER

Monday

Tuesday

Wednesday

Thursday

Friday

Saturday

Sunday

Shopping List:

_____
_____
_____
_____
_____
_____
_____
_____
_____
_____
_____
_____
_____
_____
_____
_____
_____
_____
_____
_____

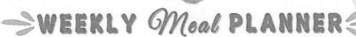

⇒WEEKLY *Meal* PLANNER⇐

Monday

Tuesday

Wednesday

Thursday

Friday

Saturday

Sunday

Shopping List:

_____
_____
_____
_____
_____
_____
_____
_____
_____
_____
_____
_____
_____
_____
_____
_____
_____
_____
_____
_____
_____
_____

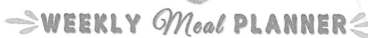

WEEKLY *Meal* PLANNER

Monday

Tuesday

Wednesday

Thursday

Friday

Saturday

Sunday

Shopping List:

_____
_____
_____
_____
_____
_____
_____
_____
_____
_____
_____
_____
_____
_____
_____
_____
_____
_____
_____

WEEKLY *Meal* PLANNER

Monday

Tuesday

Wednesday

Thursday

Friday

Saturday

Sunday

Shopping List:

_____
_____
_____
_____
_____
_____
_____
_____
_____
_____
_____
_____
_____
_____
_____
_____
_____
_____
_____
_____
_____

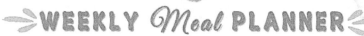

WEEKLY *Meal* PLANNER

Monday

Tuesday

Wednesday

Thursday

Friday

Saturday

Sunday

Shopping List:
_____
_____
_____
_____
_____
_____
_____
_____
_____
_____
_____
_____
_____
_____
_____
_____
_____
_____
_____
_____
_____
_____

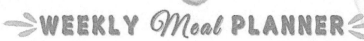

WEEKLY *Meal* PLANNER

Monday

Tuesday

Wednesday

Thursday

Friday

Saturday

Sunday

Shopping List:

_____
_____
_____
_____
_____
_____
_____
_____
_____
_____
_____
_____
_____
_____
_____
_____
_____
_____
_____

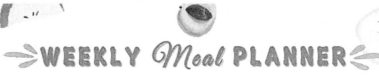

WEEKLY *Meal* PLANNER

Monday

Tuesday

Wednesday

Thursday

Friday

Saturday

Sunday

Shopping List:

_____

_____

_____

_____

_____

_____

_____

_____

_____

_____

_____

_____

_____

_____

_____

_____

_____

_____

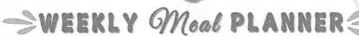

WEEKLY *Meal* PLANNER

Monday

Tuesday

Wednesday

Thursday

Friday

Saturday

Sunday

Shopping List:

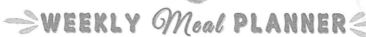 WEEKLY *Meal* PLANNER

Monday

Tuesday

Wednesday

Thursday

Friday

Saturday

Sunday

Shopping List:

_____
_____
_____
_____
_____
_____
_____
_____
_____
_____
_____
_____
_____
_____
_____
_____
_____
_____
_____
_____
_____

WEEKLY *Meal* PLANNER

Monday

Tuesday

Wednesday

Thursday

Friday

Saturday

Sunday

Shopping List:

_____
_____
_____
_____
_____
_____
_____
_____
_____
_____
_____
_____
_____
_____
_____
_____
_____
_____
_____
_____
_____
_____

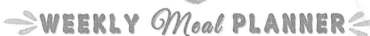

WEEKLY *Meal* PLANNER

Monday

Tuesday

Wednesday

Thursday

Friday

Saturday

Sunday

Shopping List:

_____
_____
_____
_____
_____
_____
_____
_____
_____
_____
_____
_____
_____
_____
_____
_____
_____
_____
_____
_____
_____

WEEKLY 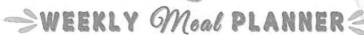 Meal PLANNER

Monday

Tuesday

Wednesday

Thursday

Friday

Saturday

Sunday

Shopping List:

_____
_____
_____
_____
_____
_____
_____
_____
_____
_____
_____
_____
_____
_____
_____
_____
_____
_____
_____

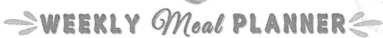

WEEKLY *Meal* PLANNER

Monday

Tuesday

Wednesday

Thursday

Friday

Saturday

Sunday

Shopping List:

_____
_____
_____
_____
_____
_____
_____
_____
_____
_____
_____
_____
_____
_____
_____
_____
_____
_____
_____
_____
_____

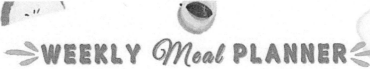

WEEKLY *Meal* PLANNER

Monday

Tuesday

Wednesday

Thursday

Friday

Saturday

Sunday

Shopping List:

_____
_____
_____
_____
_____
_____
_____
_____
_____
_____
_____
_____
_____
_____
_____
_____
_____
_____
_____
_____
_____
_____
_____

WEEKLY *Meal* PLANNER

Monday

Tuesday

Wednesday

Thursday

Friday

Saturday

Sunday

Shopping List:

WEEKLY *Meal* PLANNER

Monday

Tuesday

Wednesday

Thursday

Friday

Saturday

Sunday

Shopping List:

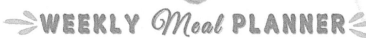

WEEKLY *Meal* PLANNER

Monday	Shopping List:
Tuesday	
Wednesday	
Thursday	
Friday	
Saturday	
Sunday	

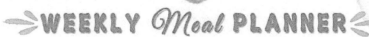

WEEKLY *Meal* PLANNER

Monday

Tuesday

Wednesday

Thursday

Friday

Saturday

Sunday

Shopping List:

_____
_____
_____
_____
_____
_____
_____
_____
_____
_____
_____
_____
_____
_____
_____
_____
_____
_____
_____
_____
_____

⇒WEEKLY *Meal* PLANNER⇐

Monday

Tuesday

Wednesday

Thursday

Friday

Saturday

Sunday

Shopping List:

_____
_____
_____
_____
_____
_____
_____
_____
_____
_____
_____
_____
_____
_____
_____
_____
_____
_____
_____
_____
_____

WEEKLY Meal PLANNER

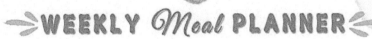

Monday

Tuesday

Wednesday

Thursday

Friday

Saturday

Sunday

Shopping List:

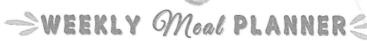

WEEKLY Meal PLANNER

Monday

Tuesday

Wednesday

Thursday

Friday

Saturday

Sunday

Shopping List:

WEEKLY *Meal* PLANNER

Monday

Tuesday

Wednesday

Thursday

Friday

Saturday

Sunday

Shopping List:

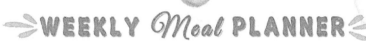

WEEKLY *Meal* PLANNER

Monday

Tuesday

Wednesday

Thursday

Friday

Saturday

Sunday

Shopping List:

_____

_____

_____

_____

_____

_____

_____

_____

_____

_____

_____

_____

_____

_____

_____

_____

_____

_____

_____

_____

_____

_____

_____

_____

Printed in Great Britain
by Amazon

45943298R00076